21 DAY SMOOTHIE CHALLENGE

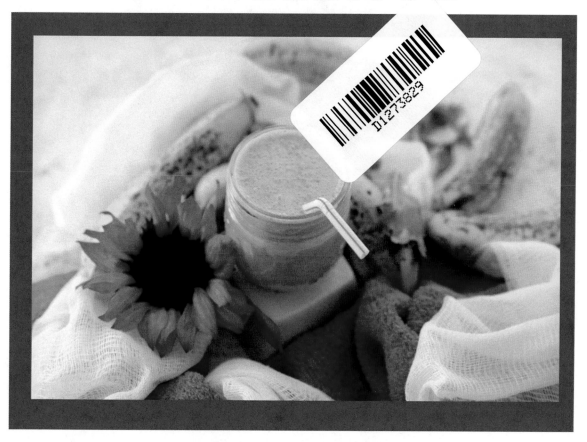

Written, Photographed and Designed by Rawnda Flowers
Copyright © February 2021

Print version available via AMAZON
ISBN: 9798709395060

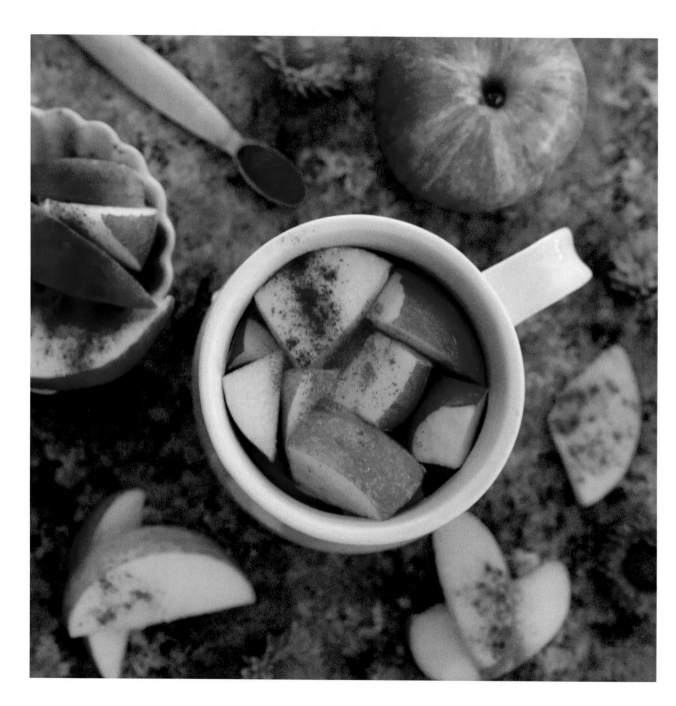

WELCOME FRIENDS!

I am so excited for you to start this challenge! I know you can do this!

I am so passionate about this lifestyle, the raw food diet.

I know that you will enjoy the freedom that comes with this lifestyle. The freedom of no longer being addicted to foods and drinks that are no longer serving you.

If you are a raw vegan now, this smoothie challenge will boost your energy levels and give you better digestion because the food will be in a smoothie form.

If you are currently eating the standard american diet, this smoothie challenge will help to reboot your taste buds and help you transition into a raw vegan diet.

-OR-

It will help you if you are only looking to incorporate more raw foods into your diet.

WELCOME (CON'T)

This book contains:

- "My Story", telling you about my experiences on the smoothie challenge.

- "Before you start (read)". You will need to read this section before you start.

- "How to use this book" (please read).

- I will give you some ideas on how to stay on this challenge, things that helped me.

- Make sure to read all the book before starting your challenge.

- All Smoothies have the approximate macros for the Calories, Fats, Proteins and Carbs.

If you have my e-book and would like to see my latest 21 Day Smoothie Challenge, **_CLICK HERE._** If you the paperback, you can go to my YouTube Channel.

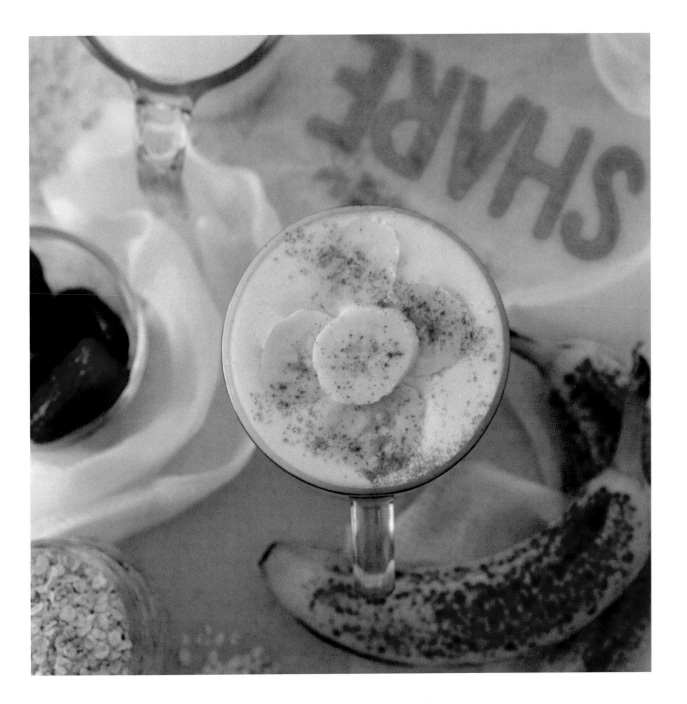

TABLE OF CONTENTS

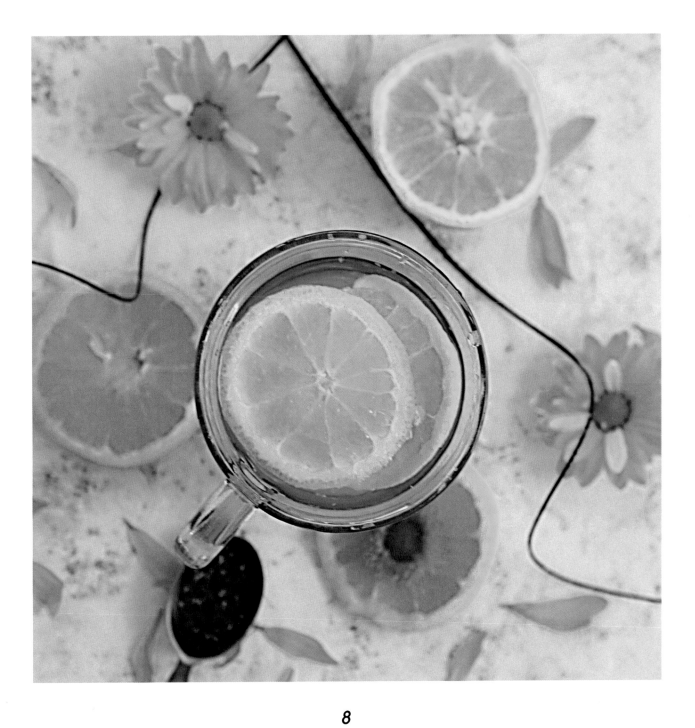

MY STORY

My name is Rawnda Flowers, I am 53 year old now in 2021.

I love to do 21 Day Smoothie Challenges because they help to reboot my whole body, my taste buds and digestive system.

Studies have shown that it takes 21 days for your taste buds to change, so if you are trying to get off the junk foods to go to a more plant based lifestyle this challenge is perfect for that.

This book is in relation to my last 21 Day Smoothie Challenge.

The last Smoothie Challenge I did was last year in 2020.

If you would like to see that challenge, I recorded my journey in those videos on my YouTube channel at Rawnda Flowers.

I created a "Playlist" called "21 Day Smoothie Challenge / Vegan", if you would like to see those videos, **CLICK HERE** if you have my e-book.

If you have the paperback, just go to my YouTube Channel.

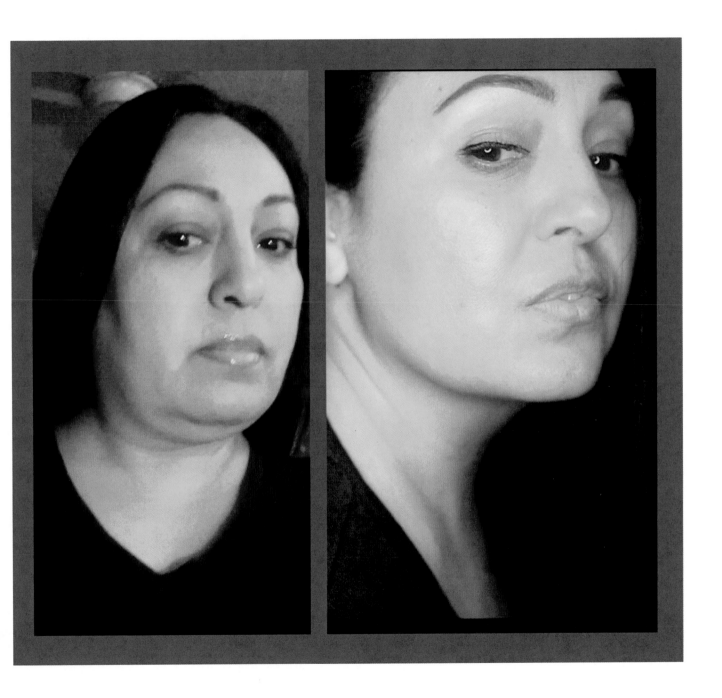

10

MY STORY (CON'T)

The reason for my last smoothie was that I was eating too many fats on my raw vegan lifestyle.

I started to gain weight and also started to have other dis-eases (meaning that my body was not at ease right now but I will be when I start the smoothie challenge) like:

My hands going numb, they really felt like they were dead (no blood circulation).

It felt like my heart was being squeezed, I thought I was going to have a heart attack.

My knee pain increased because of all the weight I gained.

I had a hard time falling asleep at night and then I would wake-up in the middle of the night and couldn't go back to bed. So I did not sleep.

I felt tired all the time, had no energy.

Had no motivation to do anything and the list goes on and on.

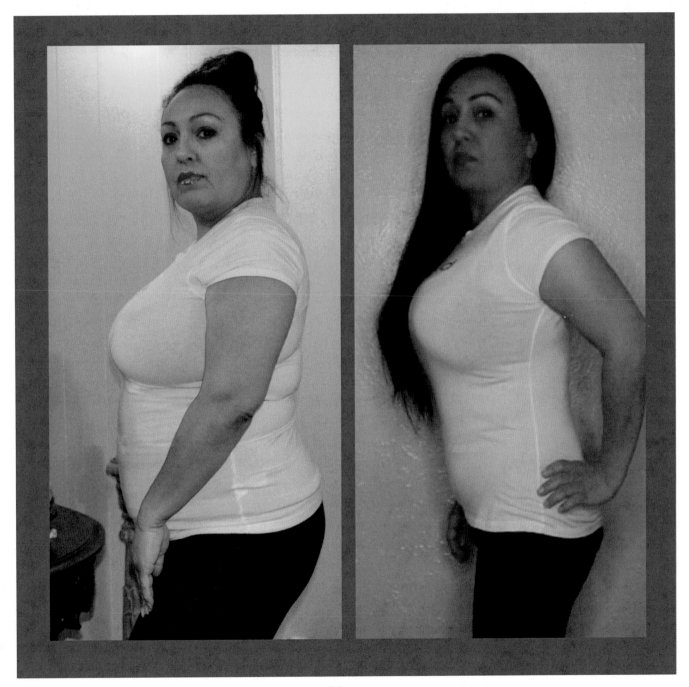

MY STORY(CON'T)

This 21 Day Smoothie Challenge was no disappointment, as soon as I started I felt amazing and had more energy.

There was a day, I believe it was the second day when I felt a little tired but then that went aways and the energy was back.

After about a week my hands were alive again, meaning that they no longer felt dead or not getting blood circulation at night when I slept.

I started sleeping throughout the night and had a better, deeper sleep.

My knee started not to hurt anymore because I started losing weight.

I recommend that you go watch my videos for more inspiration.

If you have not had a chance to go see them here is how my weight went:

I started the challenge on April 21,2020 and my weight was 152.8 lbs.

After the first week passed, I weighed 148.4 lbs.

MY STORY(CON'T)

The second week I fell off my plan that whole week and weighed 150.6lbs so I gained about 2 pounds back.

Because I fell off my plan this whole week I was going to just quit but then I said, "NO! I'm not quitting!".

What I decided to do was just to add another week to the challenge instead and that is what I did.

Then the following week of May 11,2021 I weighed 147.0 lbs.

And then on my last week on May 18, I weights 137.4 lbs, making that a total of 15.4 lbs that I lost for doing my 21 Day Smoothie Challenge.

Remember friends that everyone is different and my results may not be your results but be patient.

May this 21 Day Smoothie Challenge give you what you want and much much more!

XOXO Rawnda Flowers

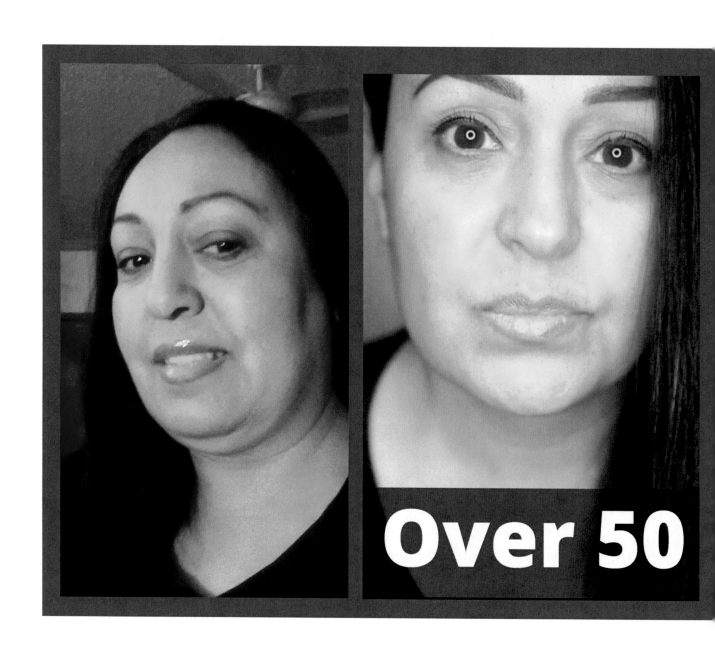

Over 50

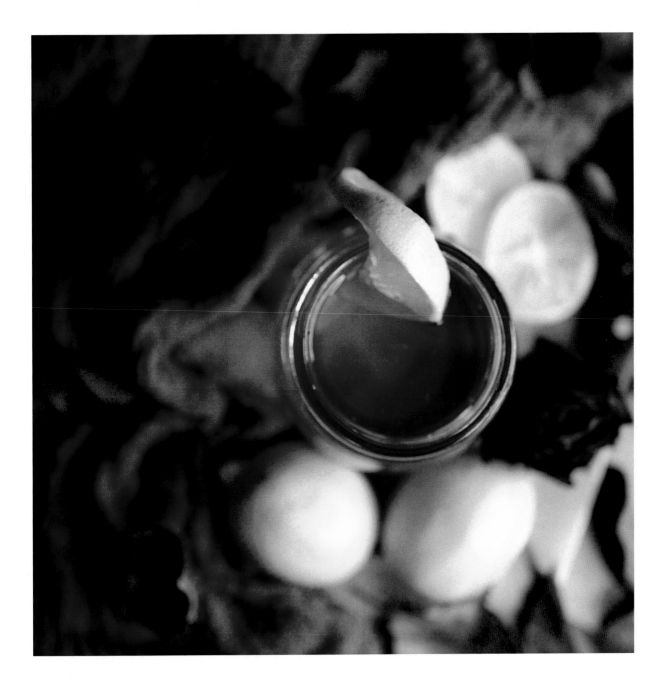

BEFORE YOU START

How to figure out how many calories you need per day:

For this 21 Day Smoothie Challenge I am doing an 80/10/10 (give or take). Basically what the 80/10/10 diet is that you eat 80% Carbs, 10% Fat and 10% protein.

There are some days that the fat, calories and protein are a little high or a little lower but for the most part they are 80/10/10.

BEFORE YOU START THIS CHALLENGE:

You will need to find out what your calculations are, find out how many calories, protein and fats you need per day to lose weight.

I was able to calculate what my Calories, protein and fats were by reading the book 80/10/10 by Doug Graham, which I bought from Amazon, if you would like to get it.

This is how I got my calculations of how many calories, fats and protein I need per day.

BEFORE YOU START (CON'T)

If you do not have the 80/10/10 Book or do not know how to get these numbers, I suggest you go to your doctor and check with him to see how many calories, fats, protein, etc. you will need in order to lose weight.

*Please read my Disclaimer, I highly recommend that you see your **doctor** if you are on any kind of medication or even if you are not.*

CRONOMETER:

Once you have figured out the amount of calories, fats and protein you need per day. You will want to use an app to calculate your food. I use Chronometer online, it's FREE.

You can track the amount of fat, calories, protein and other nutrients with this app. You want to make sure that you are getting what you need every day.

BEFORE YOU START (CON'T)

MY INTAKE FOR THIS CHALLENGE:

I am only 5 Feet tall and the amount of calories for me is anywhere from 1500 to 1650 calories per day. This is the perfect range for me.

In this book I give you a sample smoothie of what I ate with the amount of calories for me.

All you have to do is use the same fruits, veggies, etc. BUT make sure that you are adding enough calories, etc. FOR YOU.

What is in this book is the amount of calories for ME NOT YOU. Use each smoothies as a guide for your own smoothies.

I'm so excited for you to start this challenge, I know you can do this!

XOXO Rawnda Flowers

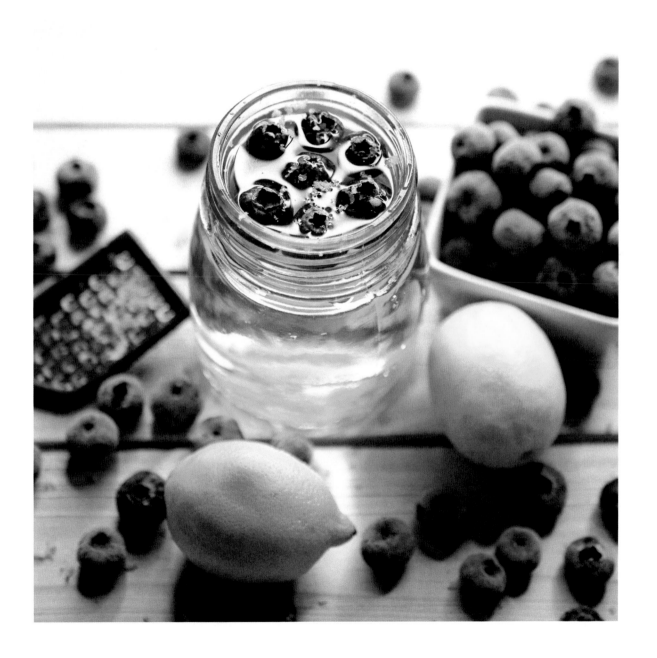

HOW TO USE THIS BOOK

This is a smoothie challenge, so basically what you are going to need is a blender, preferably a high speed blender. I have a Vitamix but you can buy another high speed blender. The Nutribullet is great.

The Vitamix is great because you will get a smooth smoothie with no chunks of pieces in the smoothie and you can warm up the smoothie in the Vitamix if you choose.

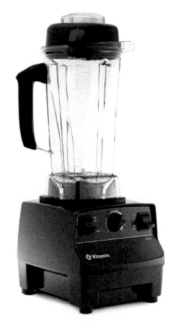

Vitamix

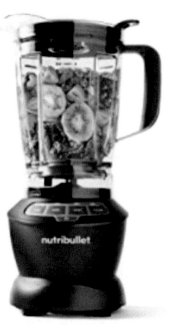

Nutribullet

HOW TO USE THIS BOOK (CON'T)

Although it is great to have a powerful blender to make the perfect smoothie, it is not necessary if you don't mind your smoothie having some chuckiness.

If you don't mind the chunkiness then you can use the blender you have.

WARM OR COLD SMOOTHIES:

If you like you can warm any smoothie or water. What you want to do is after you have made the smoothie, you can put the smoothie on a saucepan and warm it to touch, meaning that you gage it with your finger.

So as soon as you put your finger in the smoothie and it is warm then stop warming it.

The smoothie will still be raw because you can warm things up to 118 degrees without killing any of the nutrients.

HOW TO USE THIS BOOK (CON'T)

FOR THE BEST RESULTS:

For best results I suggest that the night before you write down which smoothies you are going to have for breakfast, lunch and dinner. Make sure that you have all the food you need to make your smoothies.

I know that sometimes you think you have everything you need to make a smoothie and then you look in the fridge and you realize you are missing something.

Don't let this stop you from making a smoothie, all you really need is some fruit for your calories, a little fat (chia seeds) and some greens.

Make it work, don't look for ways out but look for ways to make it work.

I know you can do this, remember the benefits that you will be getting and think of all the colorful amazing fruits that you can have and how great you feel knowing that you have accomplished your goals.

So don't forget to plan!

HOW TO USE THIS BOOK (CON'T)

Substitute Bananas:

If you don't like bananas, you can replace them with a high calorie fruit like mangos (you can google to find other high calorie fruits).

Your Appropriate Amount of Calories:

Make sure that you know how many calories YOU NEED, do not use the amount of calories that were for me.

It is very important because if you under eat you will feel tired and ravious, which will cause you to fall off your plan and you don't want that, do you!?

You also want to make sure that you are not eating too much because then you will not lose weight and feel unhealthy.

It's important that you eat the appropriate amount for you so that you can feel full and have energy during this smoothie challenge.

HOW TO USE THIS BOOK (CON'T)

Mornings

Every Morning you will have some water, you can infuse your water with fruit. I have given you several of my favorite infused water ideas along with beautiful and colorful pictures.

This is 32oz of water, which you can drink before you breakfast. If you don't finish it before you breakfast you can finish it after your breakfast.

I have given several ideas for breakfast, what I recommend is to have a breakfast of fruits or fruits and greens smoothie. All breakfast will have a little fat in the form of Chia Seeds or Flaxseed.

In this smoothie challenge you will be having fats, fats are very important. Don't think because you are having fats that you will not be able to lose weight.

You will only be having 10% of fats, that is a low but adequate amount of fat for you.

HOW TO USE THIS BOOK (CON'T)

Fats:

Fats are very important, I don't like doing a no fat smoothie challenge. In this challenge for breakfast and lunch I added fats in the form of Chia Seeds they are such a powerhouse. Some benefits I read online about Chia Seeds are:

That they are a great source of fiber
Contains essential fatty acids like Omega3 and 6
It's high in Calcium
Has 3 times more antioxidants than blueberries
Loaded with Potassium

And so much more!

*For **Breakfast, Lunch and Dinner** I have more fats in my smoothies in the form of either avocados, flaxseeds or chia seeds.*

If you do not like avocado, you can substitute it with chia seeds or flaxseeds and the same with the other fats if there is one that you do not like substitute it with another fat.

HOW TO USE THIS BOOK (CON'T)

Breakfast and Lunch

In this book there are 12 different smoothies that you can choose from for either your breakfast or lunch.

I recommend that for either your lunch or breakfast, that one of those smoothies has greens in them.

I give you a variety of ideas for the smoothies, these are some of my favorites. You can pick just a few that you like and rotate them as often as you want.

If there are only 2 or 3 that you like, that is fine, just rotate them and make sure that one of them either your breakfast or your lunch smoothie has greens in it.

If you do not like the green I have chosen then you can substitute it with other greens that you do like.

Remember it's very important to get your greens in one of those smoothies and even better if you do it for both smoothies.

HOW TO USE THIS BOOK (CON'T)

Dinner

In this book I have 10 different smoothies for dinner that you can choose from. The same goes for the dinner, if you only have a few you like then only use those few throughout the 21 Day Smoothie Challenge.

If it has greens that you do not like then substitute them with greens that you do like, for dinner make sure that you have greens in your smoothie and a fat too.

You can substitute the fats here too if you want.

There is nothing wrong if once a week you have one of the lunch or breakfast smoothies for dinner as long as you add greens to it and a fat.

HOW TO USE THIS BOOK (CON'T)

Enema

One last thing I want to talk about, I know many people don't like to talk about this but I wanted to bring it up because it may apply to you.

Some people when they first start eating more raw foods they get constipated, this is because your body is taking in so much fiber that it is just not used to it.

If this happens to be the case for you, go to your drugstore and pick up an enema bag and give yourself an enema. Once a day if needed.

If you are unsure on how to use an enema you can look at YouTube videos or consult with your doctor.

I know for me at first enemas seemed scary but once you do it one time it becomes nothing and it can relieve you of much waste and even detox symptoms if you are having some.

HOW TO USE THIS BOOK (CON'T)

READY TO START!

You are ready to start when you:

Have your amounts of calories, protein and fats for your body.
Have your blender.
Have your plan on what you are going to eat for the next day.
Have all the fruits and veggies you need for the next few days.
Have read all of the book before starting so that you know exactly what to do and how to stay motivated.

I know that you will do great! Love You!

XOXO Rawnda Flowers

TIPS & TRICKS ON STAYING MOTIVATED

STAY MOTIVATED

It's always not hard to stay motivated when starting something new and this 21 Day smoothie Challenge is no different.

Our bodies love to stay in the "COMFORT" zone.

We always try to find some reason to fall back to our old habits because they are comfortable and it's what we know BUT know that if you stay consistent you too can stay on this challenge.

With that said, I'm going to share with you some of the things I do when trying to stay motivated.

Below are some things that really helped me to stay on this smoothie challenge.

I know if I can do it, anyone can. Believe in yourself and if you fall, just get back on.

I too failed on this challenge and just extended it a week longer. So if that happens to you don be hard on yourself and just get back on.

TIPS & TRICKS ON STAYING MOTIVATED (CON'T)

Your WHY:

Motivation is a feeling which we get from our thoughts. So when you are trying to get healthy and lose weight you need a direction, something to think about that will keep you motivated.

Think about your "WHY", why are you doing this? Is it because you want to feel good and look good?

Is it because you have a special event coming?

Is it because you just lost a loved one with a certain illness and you don't want that to happen to you?

Thinking about your WHY can really help you to stay on your plan when you feel like giving up because you are tired or are just not seeing results fast as you would like it to be.

One sad thing about motivation is that MOTIVATION is fleeting. It comes and it goes. We can't always depend on it because it isn't always there.

Don't let this discourage you, this is why I always create myself a PLAN.

TIPS & TRICKS ON STAYING MOTIVATED (CON'T)

Make a Plan:

Like I mentioned, Motivation is fleeting but your PLAN isn't. Your plan is always with you when you are not feeling like staying on your road to good health.

What I did is I wrote a plan of what I will be eating and drinking every day (in this case we are making smoothies). I would do this the night before going to bed.

Example (make sure you use the appropriate amounts of calories for you):

Morning Hydration:
Lemon with Water 32oz

Breakfast:
5 Bananas, 2 dates, 2 cups of greens, chia seeds (smoothie)

Lunch:
2 Cups of Blueberries, 2 cups of greens, chia seeds (smoothie)

TIPS & TRICKS ON STAYING MOTIVATED (CON'T)

Dinner:
2 tomatoes, handful of parsley, 7 dates, 1 stalk celery, 1 carrot, piece of avocado and ½ beet (smoothie)

Once you make your plan stick to it, carry it around with you. Stick it on the fridge whatever it takes for you to see it as often as you can.

Your plan can always be with you and it will never leave you like motivation.

IMPORTANT ABOUT YOUR PLAN:

Make sure that you are drinking enough calories, make sure that you have calculated your calorie intake correctly. If you are not eating enough you will be hungry and this could cause you to fall off your plan.

I recommend that if you are feeling hungry, make yourself another smoothie and don't think that this will make you fat or not work for you.

It's better to drink another smoothie than to fall off your plan completely. You may have just calculated your calorie intake wrong or for some reason your body is needing more calories for that day.

TIPS & TRICKS ON STAYING MOTIVATED (CON'T)

Weighing yourself:

One of the biggest ways I found to keep me motivated is by NOT weighing myself everyday. I found that just weighing myself once a week is good.

If you weigh yourself everyday you will find that sometimes for days you do not lose anything and this can be discouraging.

Please know that you body knows what it is doing and it's first priority is not losing weight, it is to make you healthy and trust me the losing weight will follow.

I know some people I have worked with didn't lose but 2 pounds the first week but then the following week they lost 7 pounds.

Everyone is different and everyone's body will do what it needs to do in it's own time.

TIPS & TRICKS ON STAYING MOTIVATED (CON'T)

Watching TV:

I recommend that you do not watch TV.

I know you are probably like, "WHAT?, NO TV?"
No doubt you have noticed that when watching TV there are hundreds of commercials promoting foods and by watching those commercials you may fall off your plan.

What I recommend is if you have just regular TV, when a commercial starts walk away from the room and lower the volume so that you also not hear the commercial explaining how great that fast food item is.

If you have cable, when a commercial is coming on, just fast forward it. Another thing you can do is just watch movies with no commercials.

You can also just rent movies and fast forward if there is a food commercial in it.

By doing these things you will be more likely to stay on your plan.

TIPS & TRICKS ON STAYING MOTIVATED (CON'T)

Staying Home:

During this 21 Day Smoothie Challenge you may have the privilege of just staying home and not having to worry about others asking you why you are not eating or why you are drinking a smoothie.

BUT if you have to go somewhere, to visit a relative or a friend what I used to do is make sure I had my smoothie before I went to visit and sometimes I would even make a smoothie and take it with me. Even if this was an extra smoothie for the day, it's not something that happened often.

Don't go and visit first and then decide to have you smoothie afterwards because when you have not yet had your smoothie and you leave for the day you might start to get hungry before you know it or your family and friends might start cooking and that will make you fall off because you are not full on your smoothie.

Most of us now are able to work from home but if you have to go to a job while doing this smoothie challenge, I recommend that you buy a small cooler or just a small bag with some cooling block. You can make your smoothies in the morning for your breakfast and lunch and put those in the cooler to take to work.

TIPS & TRICKS ON STAYING MOTIVATED (CON'T)

RESULTS:

Nothing really creates MOTIVATION AND MOMENTUM like RESULTS.

No one can argue with the fact that once you start to see results from all the hard work that you are putting in you start to feel more motivated.

When you start to actually see results you start to believe even stronger that this is possible and that you can do it.

Just remember that in the beginning it is harder to stay motivated because this is something new for you or something different that you are doing to get healthy and lose weight BUT just know if you stick with it you will start to see results and the RESULTS in turn will start to motivate you.

TIPS & TRICKS ON STAYING MOTIVATED (CON'T)

The reason why I do a 21 Day Challenge is because I've read that it takes 21 days to change your taste buds.

I've also read that it only takes 10 days for your sugar craving to go away.

In my experience I have found these things to be true.

YES YOU CAN!

I JUST WANT TO LET YOU KNOW THAT I BELIEVE THAT YOU CAN DO ANYTHING THAT YOU SET YOUR MIND TO AND DON'T LET OTHERS WHO DON'T UNDERSTAND WHY YOU ARE DOING THIS CHALLENGE TO MAKE YOU FALL.

STAY TRUE TO YOURSELF.

XOXO Rawnda Flowers

MORNING

HYDRATION

MORNING HYDRATION

While we sleep our bodies are fasting (not eating mode), so in the morning to help my body flush out all the toxins I like to have a 32oz of water with lemon.

Most of the time I choose the lemon and water but other times I buy all types of fruit and infuse my water with it.

What I like to do is the night before is put some fruit in my water and leave it in the fridge. That way in the morning when I get up it's ready for me to consume.

I know a lot of people don't like drinking just water so by infusing your water with fruit it helps you to better enjoy the water. I personally do not eat the fruit in the water. Therefore I did not give you the macros for these waters.

Just remember if you do eat the fruit to calculate it in the cronometer.

MORNING HYDRATION (CON'T)

If I do not finish my water by the time I decide to drink my morning breakfast, I just finish it after breakfast.

I have provided you with 11 of my favorite morning drinks, feel free to use all of them or just pick a few you like. Wanted to make sure you get a variety.

Also remember if you want to have a warm drink you can warm these drinks to touch, meaning as soon as it is warm to your finger take it away from the stove.

Enjoy your morning hydration friends!

LEMON WATER

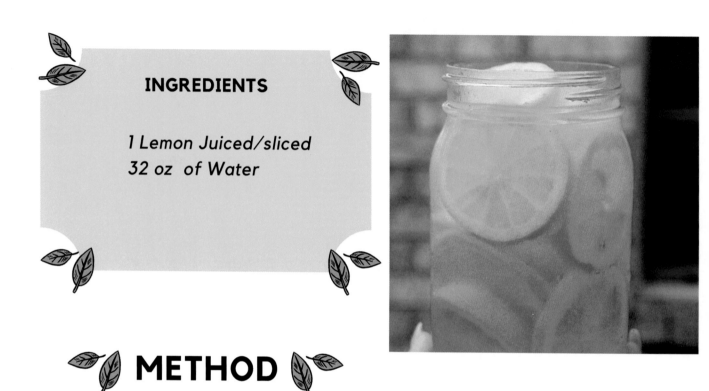

INGREDIENTS

1 Lemon Juiced/sliced
32 oz of Water

METHOD

Put all ingredients in the glass of water and Enjoy! You can do this first thing in the morning or you can do it the night before and put it in the fridge.

Note: If you would like it warm, you can warm it to touch. As long as you don't warm it higher than 118 degrees it's still raw.

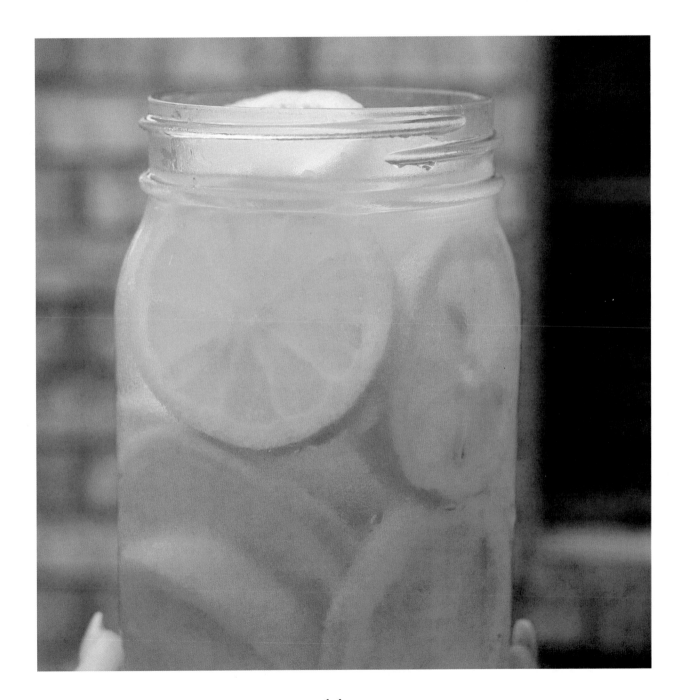

44

ORANGE CHIA

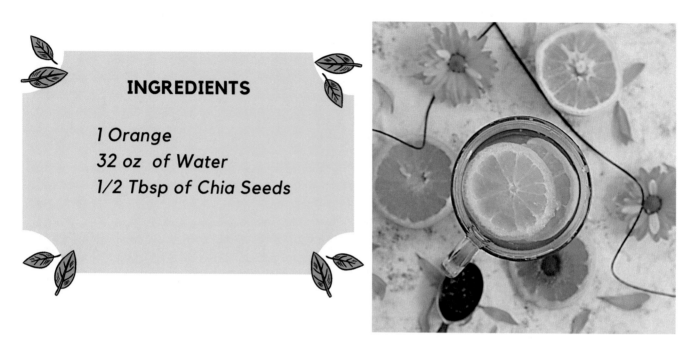

INGREDIENTS

1 Orange
32 oz of Water
1/2 Tbsp of Chia Seeds

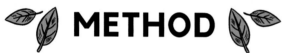

METHOD

Put all ingredients in the glass of water and Enjoy! You can do this first thing in the morning or you can do it the night before and put it in the fridge.

Note: If you would like it warm, you can warm it to touch. As long as you don't warm it higher than 118 degrees it's still raw.

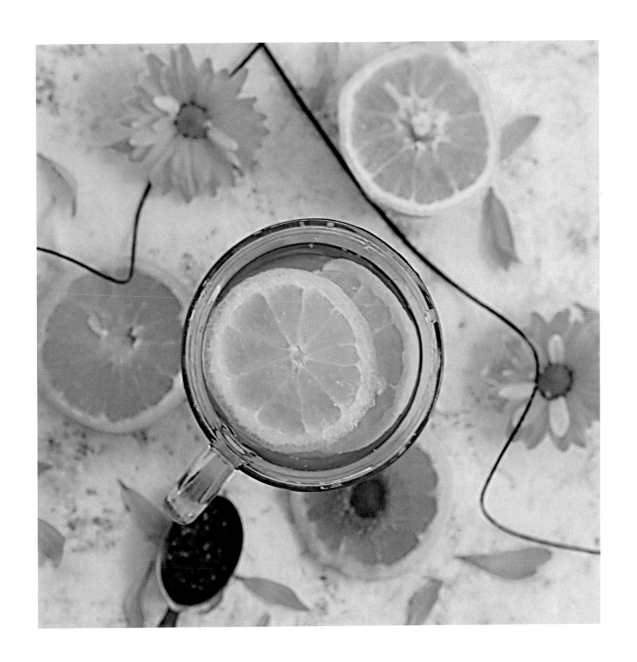

CINNAPPLE CANDY

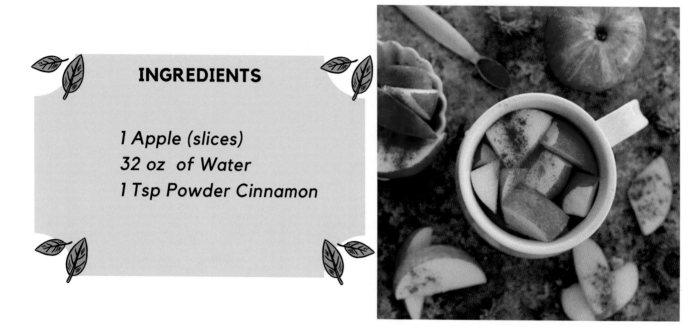

INGREDIENTS

1 Apple (slices)
32 oz of Water
1 Tsp Powder Cinnamon

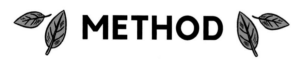 # METHOD

Put all ingredients in the glass of water and Enjoy! You can do this first thing in the morning or you can do it the night before and put it in the fridge.

Note: If you would like it warm, you can warm it to touch. As long as you don't warm it higher than 118 degrees it's still raw.

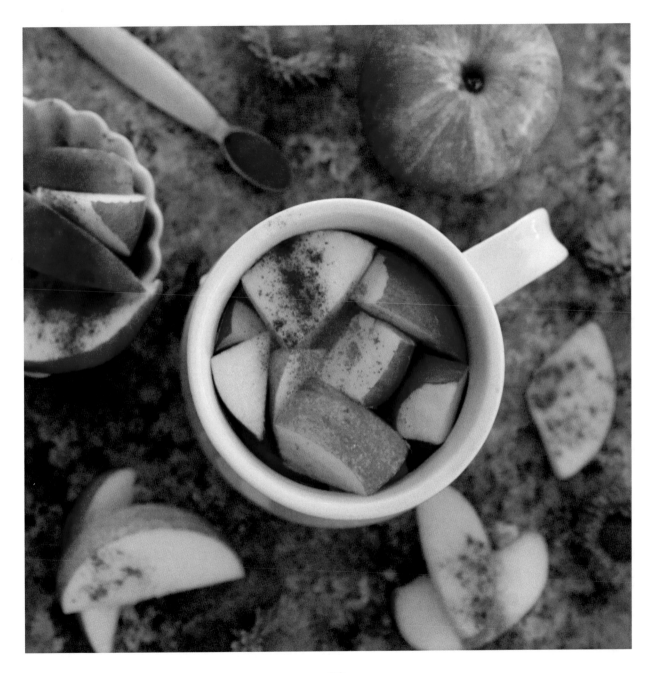

WATERMELON SUN

INGREDIENTS

1/2 Lemon sliced
3 Small slices of Watermelon
A pinch of Edible Flowers
32 oz of Water

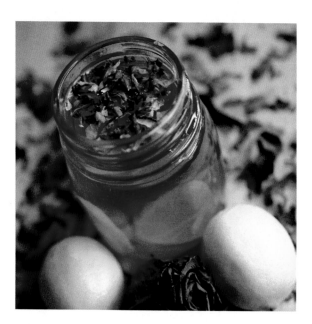

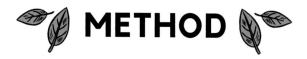 ## METHOD

Put all ingredients in the glass of water and Enjoy! You can do this first thing in the morning or you can do it the night before and put it in the fridge.

Note: If you would like it warm, you can warm it to touch. As long as you don't warm it higher than 118 degrees it's still raw.

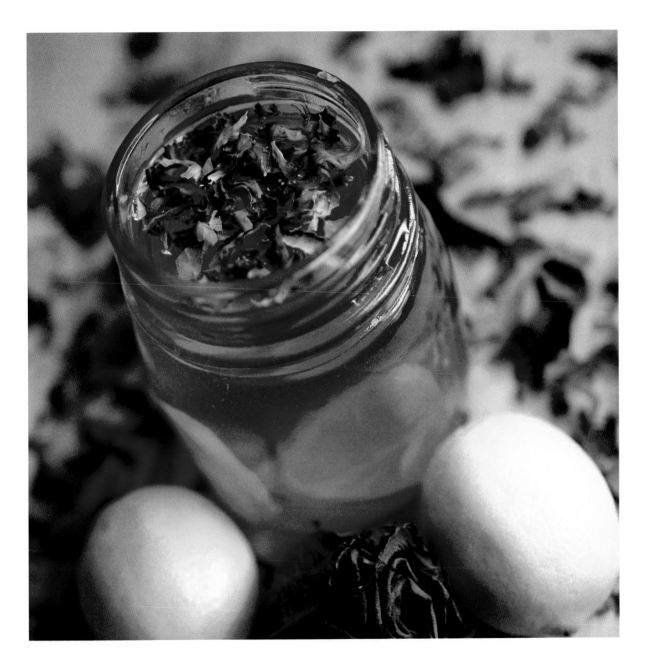

TINY BLISS TANGERINE

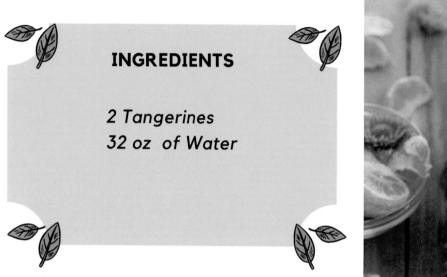

INGREDIENTS

2 Tangerines
32 oz of Water

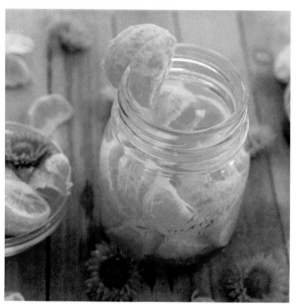

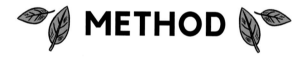 **METHOD**

Put all ingredients in the glass of water and Enjoy! You can do this first thing in the morning or you can do it the night before and put it in the fridge.

Note: If you would like it warm, you can warm it to touch. As long as you don't warm it higher than 118 degrees it's still raw.

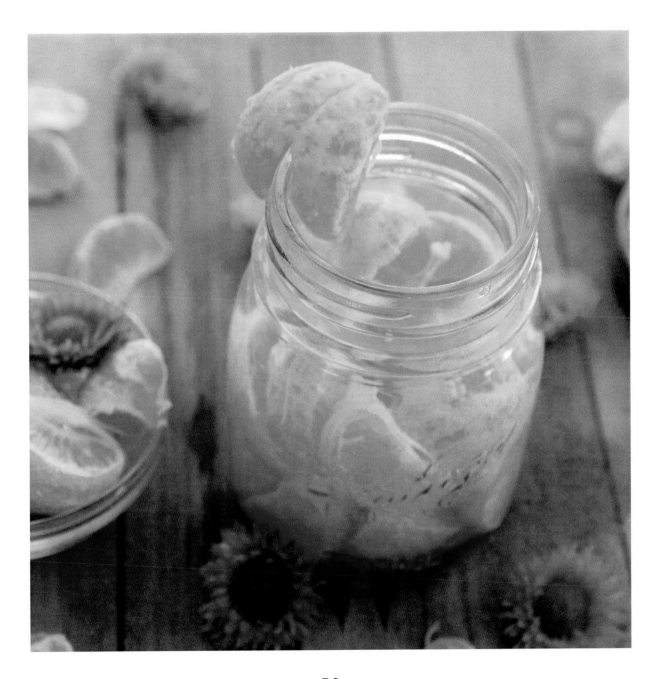

LEMON & CUCUMBER

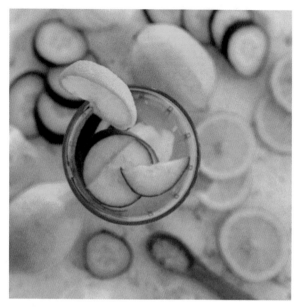

INGREDIENTS

1 Lemon
1/2 Cucumber
Pinch of Himalayan Salt
32 oz of Water

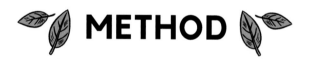 **METHOD**

Put all ingredients in the glass of water and Enjoy! You can do this first thing in the morning or you can do it the night before and put it in the fridge.

Note: If you would like it warm, you can warm it to touch. As long as you don't warm it higher than 118 degrees it's still raw.

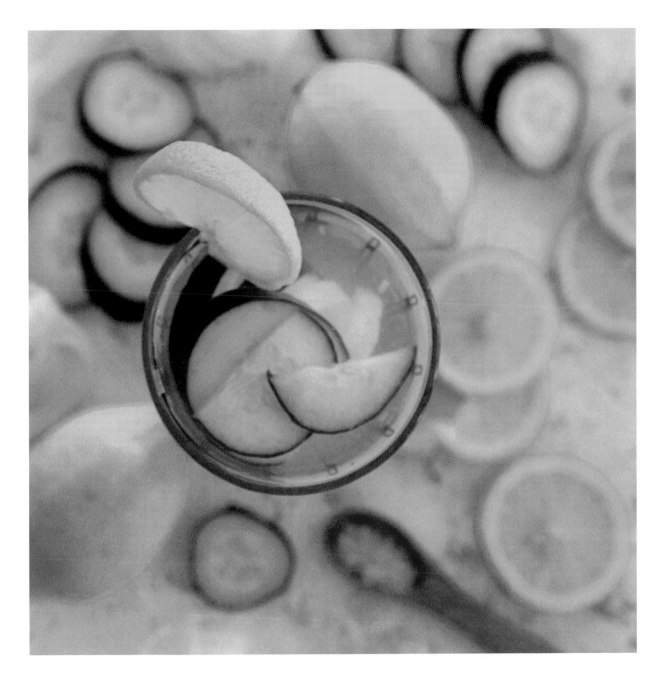

54

RED LEMON JUICE

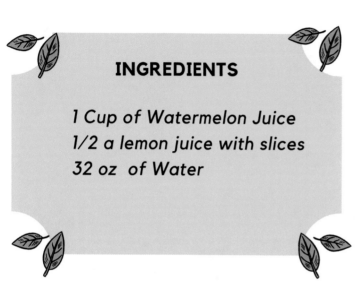

INGREDIENTS

1 Cup of Watermelon Juice
1/2 a lemon juice with slices
32 oz of Water

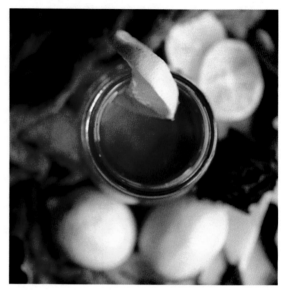

METHOD

Put all ingredients in the glass of water and Enjoy! You can do this first thing in the morning or you can do it the night before and put it in the fridge.

Note: If you would like it warm, you can warm it to touch. As long as you don't warm it higher than 118 degrees it's still raw.

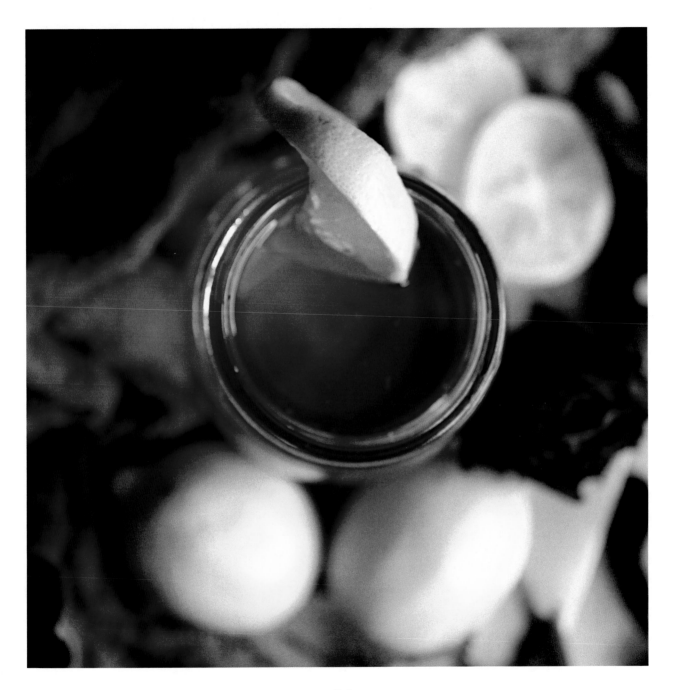

BLUEBERRY DREAMS

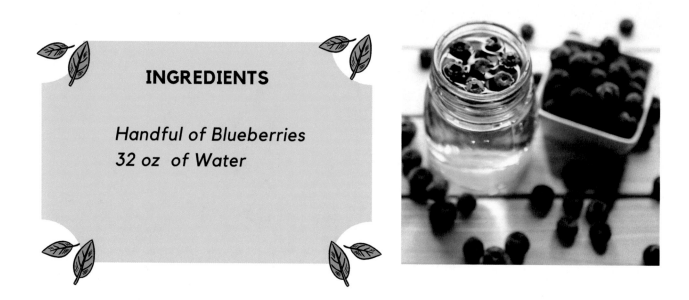

INGREDIENTS

Handful of Blueberries
32 oz of Water

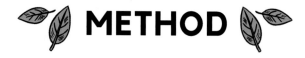 ## METHOD

Put all ingredients in the glass of water and Enjoy! You can do this first thing in the morning or you can do it the night before and put it in the fridge.

Note: If you would like it warm, you can warm it to touch. As long as you don't warm it higher than 118 degrees it's still raw.

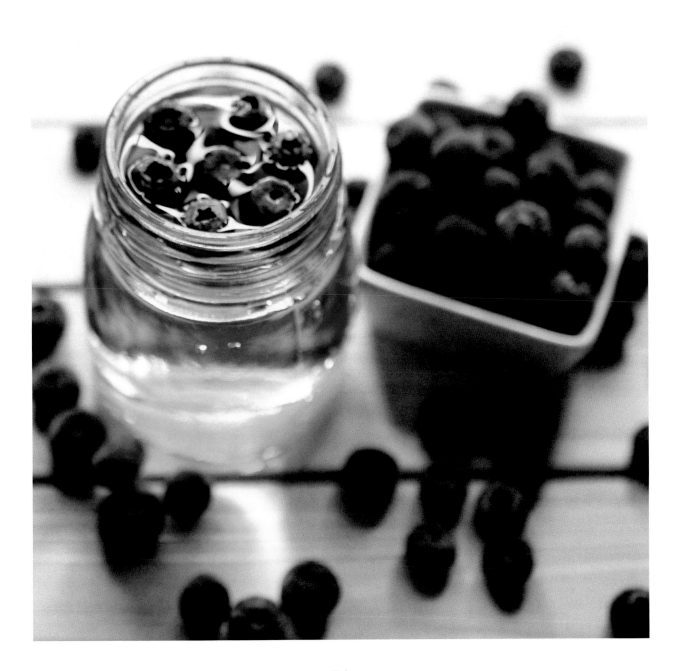

CUCUMBER TANG

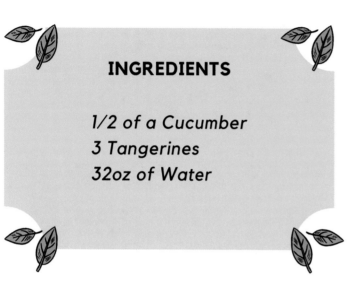

INGREDIENTS

1/2 of a Cucumber
3 Tangerines
32oz of Water

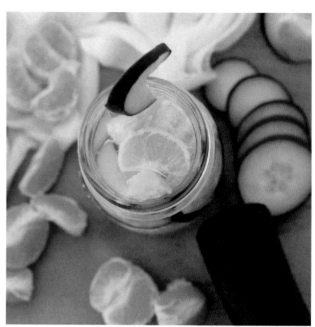

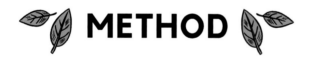 ## METHOD

Put all ingredients in the glass of water and Enjoy! You can do this first thing in the morning or you can do it the night before and put it in the fridge.

Note: If you would like it warm, you can warm it to touch. As long as you don't warm it higher than 118 degrees it's still raw.

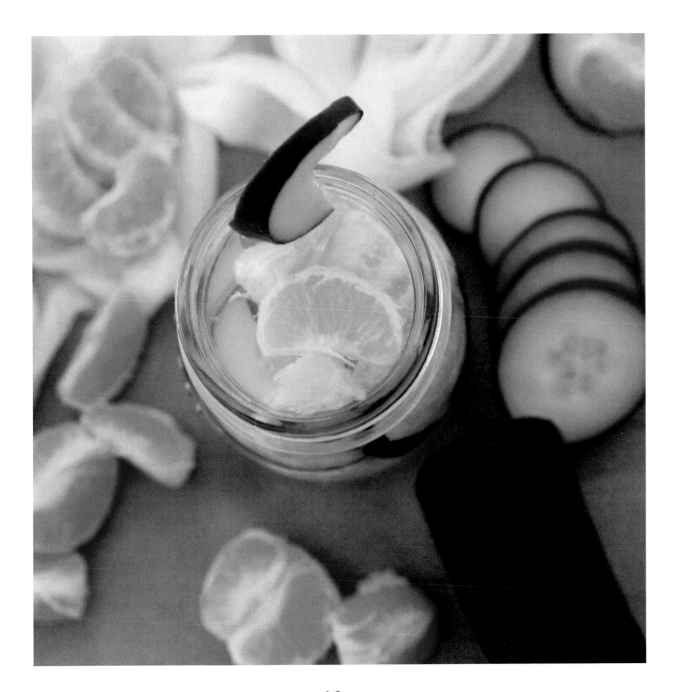

BLUE BEAUTY BERRIES

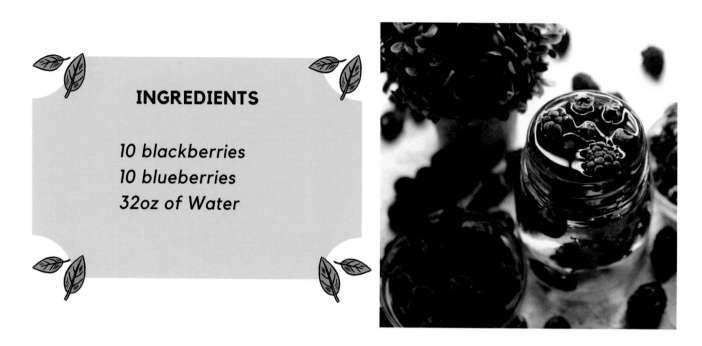

INGREDIENTS

10 blackberries
10 blueberries
32oz of Water

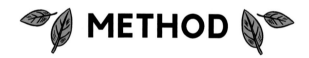 ## METHOD

Put all ingredients in the glass of water and Enjoy! You can do this first thing in the morning or you can do it the night before and put it in the fridge.

Note: If you would like it warm, you can warm it to touch. As long as you don't warm it higher than 118 degrees it's still raw.

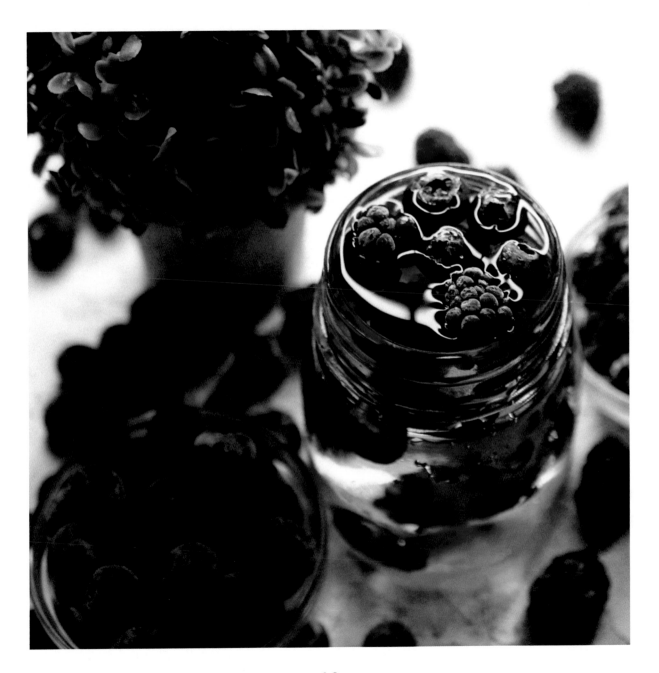

ORANGE & LEMON

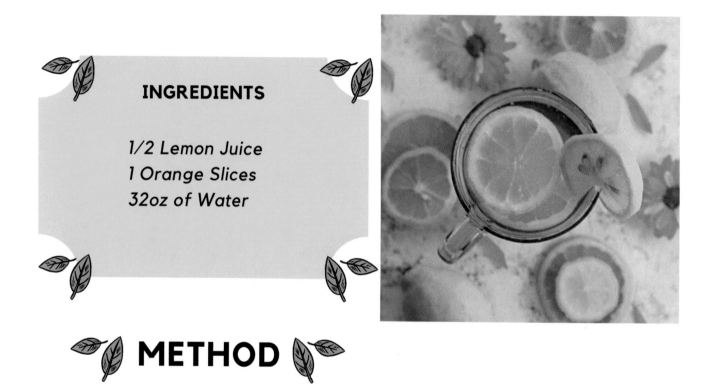

INGREDIENTS

1/2 Lemon Juice
1 Orange Slices
32oz of Water

METHOD

Put all ingredients in the glass of water and Enjoy! You can do this first thing in the morning or you can do it the night before and put it in the fridge.

Note: If you would like it warm, you can warm it to touch. As long as you don't warm it higher than 118 degrees it's still raw.

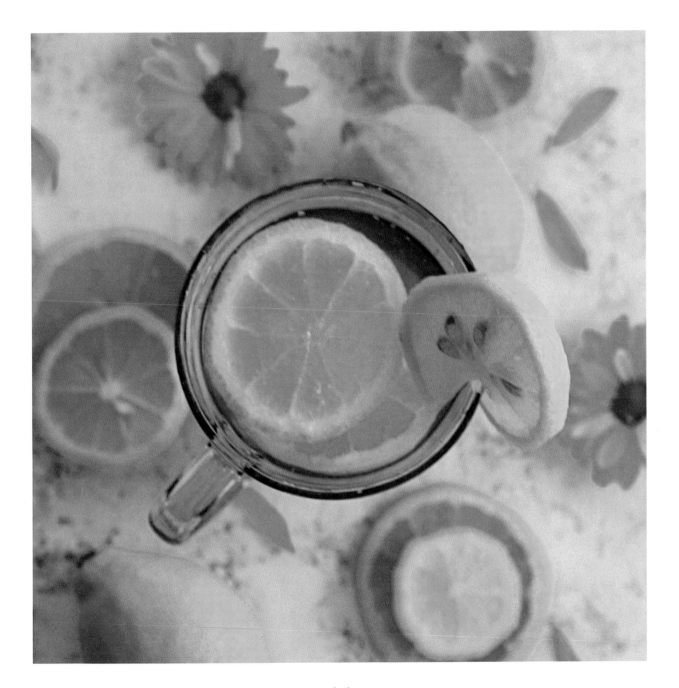

BLUEBERRY SUNSHINE

INGREDIENTS

1/2 Lemon Juice
Handful of blueberries
32oz of Water

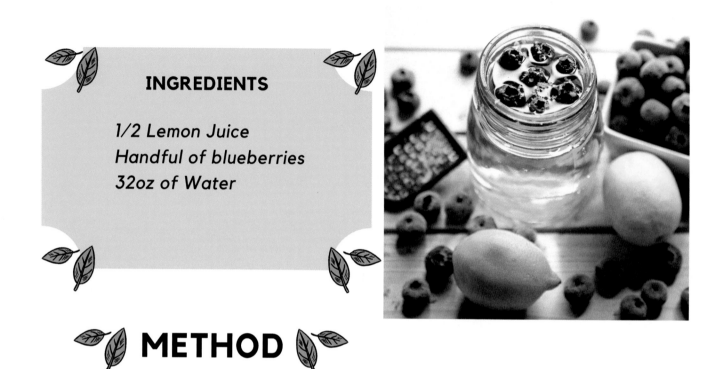

METHOD

Put all ingredients in the glass of water and Enjoy! You can do this first thing in the morning or you can do it the night before and put it in the fridge.

Note: If you would like it warm, you can warm it to touch. As long as you don't warm it higher than 118 degrees it's still raw.

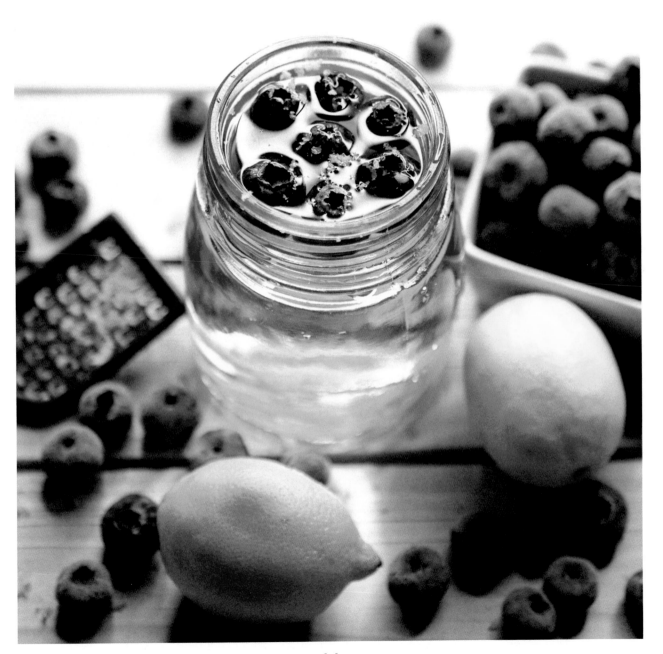

BREAKFAST
&
LUNCH

BREAKFAST
&
LUNCH

For breakfast I like to have a fruit smoothie to give me the energy I need until my lunch. Sometimes in these breakfast smoothies I do like to add greens to them.

I have provided you with 12 of my favorite smoothies that I have for both breakfast and lunch.

A few of these smoothies don't have greens in them, I recommend that you have those for breakfast but maybe once a week you can have it for lunch.

The important thing is to make sure that one of your smoothies has GREENS in it, either the breakfast or the lunch.

Also, while I am creating this book it is winter here in Texas and pretty cold, so if it is cold where you are right now or when you decide to take the challenge, remember that you can warm these smoothies to touch.

Enjoy your Breakfast and Lunches!!

BANANA SMOOTHIE

INGREDIENTS

3 Medium Bananas
2 Medjool Dates
3 Tbsp Chia Seeds
2 Cups Spinach
2 Cups of Water

APPROXIMATE MICRONUTRITION BREAKDOWN

Total Calories: 510
Total Fat: 4.5g
Total Protein: 8.1g
Total Carbs: 123.2g

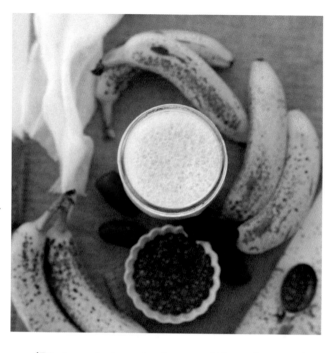

(Picture taken before adding Greens)

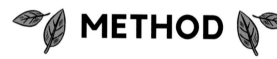 **METHOD**

In a high speed blender, blend all the bananas, dates and 2 cups of spinach with 2 cups of water and blend until the smoothie is smooth.

Note: If you would like it to be thicker add less water or if you want it more liquidy add more water.

OATMEAL SMOOTHIE

INGREDIENTS

2 Medium Bananas
3 Medjool Dates
2 Tbsp of Oats
1 Tsp of Flaxseeds
1 Tsp Ground Cinnamon
1 Cups of Water

APPROXIMATE MICRONUTRITION BREAKDOWN

Total Calories: 558
Total Fat: 4.6g
Total Protein: 7.0g
Total Carbs: 136.8g

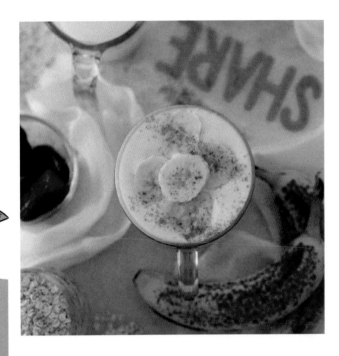

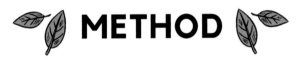 **METHOD**

In a high speed blender, blend 1 bananas, dates, cinnamon, Oats, flaxseeds and almond milk and blend until the smoothie is smooth. Pour in a glass and cut 2nd banana into quarters, put on top of smoothie and sprinkle cinnamon and Enjoy!

Note: Make sure you get Raw Oatmeal that is gluten free certified.

PINK DRAGON FRUIT

INGREDIENTS

4 Medium Bananas
1 Pack of Dragon Fruit *
2 Tbsp of Chia seeds
2 Cups water

APPROXIMATE MICRONUTRITION BREAKDOWN

Total Calories: 577
Total Fat: 7.7g
Total Protein: 9.5g
Total Carbs: 129.2g

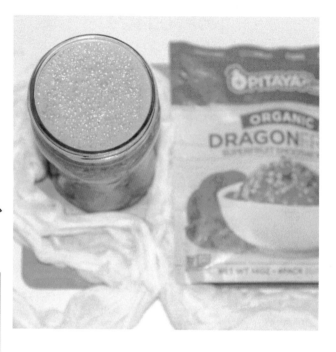

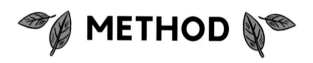 **METHOD**

In a high speed blender, blend the bananas, kale, acai and 2 cup of water, until smooth. Add chia seeds to smoothie after you blend.

Note: If you would like it to be thicker add less water or if you want it more liquidy add more water. ***You can find Dragon Fruit packs at Whole Foods.***

STRAWBERRY SMOOTHIE

INGREDIENTS

1 Cup of Strawberries
3 Medjool Dates
2 Bananas
1 Cup Water
2 Tbsp of Chia Seeds
1 Cup of Arugula

APPROXIMATE MICRONUTRITION BREAKDOWN

Total Calories: 589
Total Fat: 7.4g
Total Protein: 8.6g
Total Carbs: 137.2g

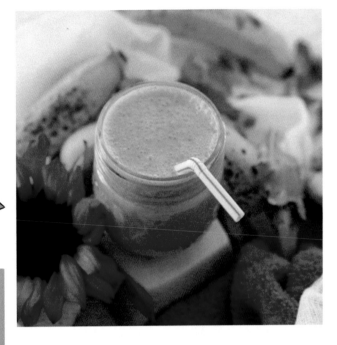

(Picture taken before adding the greens)

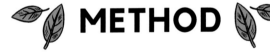 **METHOD**

In a high speed blender, blend the bananas, dates, strawberries, 1 cup of vanilla milk, 1 cup of water, chia seeds and the arugula and blend until the smoothie is smooth.

Note: *If you would like it to be thicker add less water or if you want it more liquidy add more water.*

GRAPE BUBBLE GUM

INGREDIENTS

2 Cups of Bubble Gum Grapes
3 Dates
2 Tbsp of Chia Seeds
1 Cup of baby Spinach
2 Cups of water

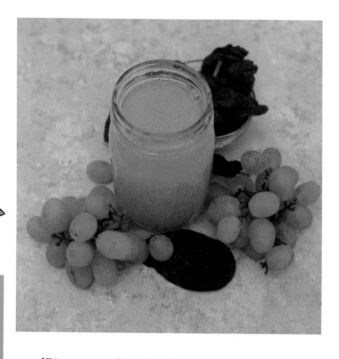

(Picture taken before adding Greens)

APPROXIMATE MICRONUTRITION BREAKDOWN

Total Calories: 512
Total Fat: 6.9g
Total Protein: 7.6g
Total Carbs: 118.2g

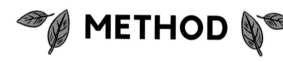 METHOD

In a high speed blender, blend the grapes, dates, spinach, and 2 cup of water, until smooth. Add chia seeds to smoothie after you blend.

Note: *If you would like it to be thicker add less water or if you want it more liquidy add more water.*

PERSIMMONS SMOOTHIE

INGREDIENTS

2 Cups of Persimmons
4 Dates
2 Tbsp of Chia Seeds
1 Cups of water

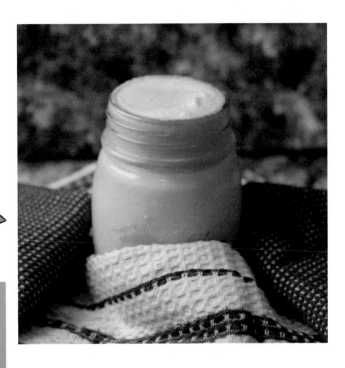

APPROXIMATE MICRONUTRITION BREAKDOWN

Total Calories: 561
Total Fat: 6.8g
Total Protein: 6.7g
Total Carbs: 132.9g

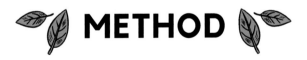 **METHOD**

In a high speed blender, blend the Persimmons, dates, almond milk and 1 cup of water, until smooth. Add chia seeds to smoothie after you blend.

Note: *If you would like it to be thicker add less water or if you want it more liquidy add more water.*

FAIRY CHERRY SMOOTHIE

INGREDIENTS

2 Cups of Cherries
5 Dates
2 Tbsp of Chia Seeds
2 Cups of water

APPROXIMATE MICRONUTRITION BREAKDOWN

Total Calories: 559
Total Fat: 2.8g
Total Protein: 6.5g
Total Carbs: 142.1g

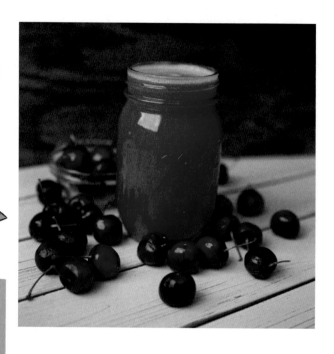

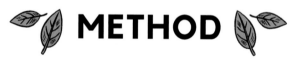 **METHOD**

In a high speed blender, blend the cherries, dates and 2 cup of water, until smooth. Add chia seeds to smoothie after you blend.

Note: *If you would like it to be thicker add less water or if you want it more liquidy add more water.*

PINEAPPLE SMOOTHIE

INGREDIENTS

2 Cups of Pineapple
5 Dates
2 Tbsp of Chia Seeds
1 Cups of water

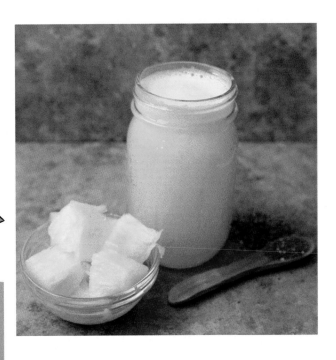

APPROXIMATE MICRONUTRITION BREAKDOWN

Total Calories: 530
Total Fat: 2.6g
Total Protein: 5.1g
Total Carbs: 136.1g

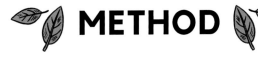 **METHOD**

In a high speed blender, blend the pineapples, dates and 1 cup of water, until smooth. Add chia seeds to smoothie after you blend.

Note: *If you would like it to be thicker add less water or if you want it more liquidy add more water.*

MANGO SMOOTHIE

INGREDIENTS

2 Cups of Mangos
3 Dates
2 Tbsp of Chia Seeds
1 Cup of Spinach
1 Cups of water

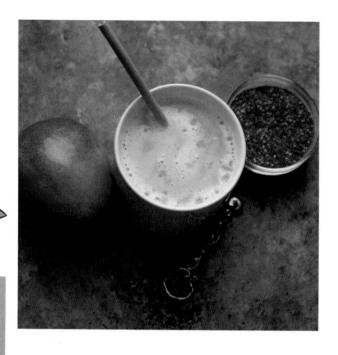

APPROXIMATE
MICRONUTRITION BREAKDOWN

Total Calories: 514
Total Fat: 4.0g
Total Protein: 7.0g
Total Carbs: 126.6g

(Picture taken before adding Greens)

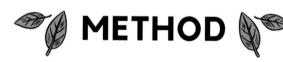

METHOD

In a high speed blender, blend the mangos, dates, spinach and 1 cup of water, until smooth. Add chia seeds to smoothie after you blend.

Note: *If you would like it to be thicker add less water or if you want it more liquidy add more water.*

BLACKBERRY SMOOTHIE

INGREDIENTS

2 Cups of Blackberries
4 Dates
2 Tbsp of Chia Seeds
2 Cups of water

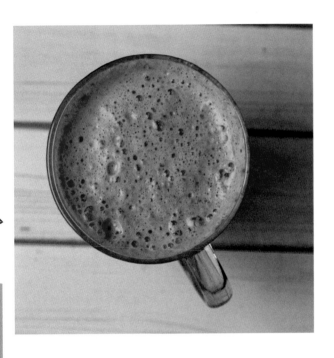

APPROXIMATE
MICRONUTRITION BREAKDOWN

Total Calories: 598
Total Fat: 9.2g
Total Protein: 7.0g
Total Carbs: 136.4g

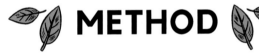 **METHOD**

In a high speed blender, blend the blackberries, dates, almond milk and 1 cup of water, until smooth. Add chia seeds to smoothie after you blend.

Note: *If you would like it to be thicker add less water or if you want it more liquidy add more water.*

MIXED GREEN SMOOTHIE

INGREDIENTS

4 Bananas
2 Cups Mixed Greens
2 Tbsp of Chia Seeds
2 Cups of water

APPROXIMATE MICRONUTRITION BREAKDOWN

Total Calories: 536
Total Fat: 8.0g
Total Protein: 10.1g
Total Carbs: 119.8g

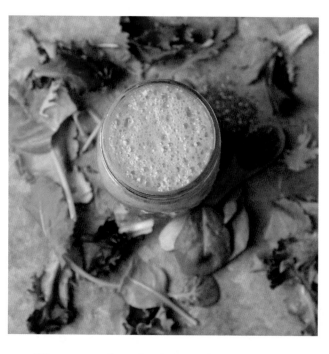

(Picture taken before adding Greens)

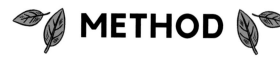 ## METHOD

In a high speed blender, blend the bananas, mix greens and 2 cup of water, until smooth. Add chia seeds to smoothie after you blend.

Note: *If you would like it to be thicker add less water or if you want it more liquidy add more water.*

ACAI SMOOTHIE

INGREDIENTS

4 Bananas
1 Pack of Acai *
2 Cups of Baby Kale
2 Tbsp of Chia Seeds
2 Cups of water

APPROXIMATE
MICRONUTRITION BREAKDOWN

Total Calories: 672
Total Fat: 19.2g
Total Protein: 11.6g
Total Carbs: 132.9g

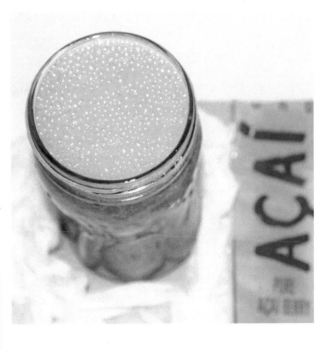

(Picture taken before adding Greens)

 METHOD

In a high speed blender, blend the bananas, kale, acai and 2 cup of water, until smooth. Add chia seeds to smoothie after you blend.

*Note: If you would like it to be thicker add less water or if you want it more liquidy add more water. **You can find ACAI packs at Whole Foods.***

DINNER

DINNER

Raw smoothies for Dinner. These smoothies are fresh, delicious, and healthy. These raw food smoothies are easy to make and fast.

I have given you 10 different smoothies to choose from, when on my 21 Day Smoothie Challenge I only really pick two to three different ones and stick with that but you can do all of them or even only one and do that for the whole 21 days (just make sure it has greens in it). It's all up to you.

Dinner is where I make sure I get more greens and fats, not overly but my appropriate amount. Make sure to go to Cronometer to make sure you are meeting your requirements.

One of my favorite smoothies is the V8 smoothie, I really think this is so delicious, filling and easy to make. It's up to you, which smoothies you want to use.

Enjoy!
Rawnda Flowers

BUTTERNUT SMOOTHIE

INGREDIENTS

2 Cups of Butternut Squash
1 Tbsp of Chia Seeds
2 Cups of Baby Spinach
5 Dates
2 Cups of water

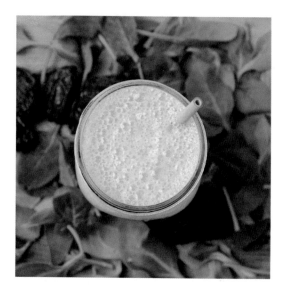

APPROXIMATE
MICRONUTRITION BREAKDOWN

Total Calories: 559
Total Fat: 3.9g
Total Protein: 9.2g
Total Carbs: 139.4g

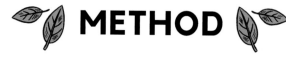 **METHOD**

In a high speed blender, blend all the ingredients until smooth. Add 1 Tbsp of chia seeds to smoothie after you blend.

Note: *If you would like it to be thicker add less water or if you want it more liquidy add more water.*

APPLE CINNAMON PIE

INGREDIENTS

3 Bananas

2 Dates

1 Apple

1 Tbsp of Cinnamon

2 Cups of Mixed Greens

2 Cups of water

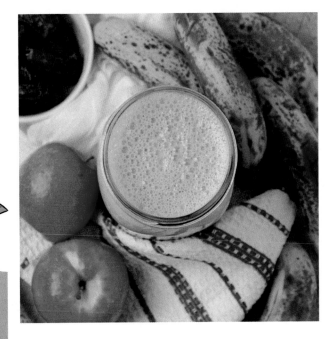

APPROXIMATE MICRONUTRITION BREAKDOWN

Total Calories: 629

Total Fat: 5.0g

Total Protein: 8.8g

Total Carbs: 156.0g

 METHOD

In a high speed blender, blend all the ingredients until smooth. Add 1 Tbsp of chia seeds to smoothie after you blend.

Note: *If you would like it to be thicker add less water or if you want it more liquidy add more water.*

GREEN VIBRANCE

INGREDIENTS

4 Bananas
1 Dates
2 Cups of Mixed Greens
2 Tbsp of Avocado
2 Cups of water

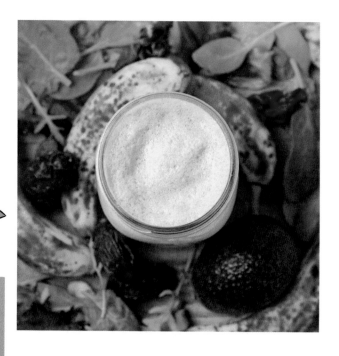

APPROXIMATE
MICRONUTRITION BREAKDOWN

Total Calories: 554
Total Fat: 6.3g
Total Protein: 7.8g
Total Carbs: 131.8g

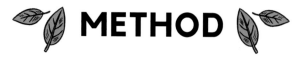 **METHOD**

In a high speed blender, blend all the ingredients until smooth. Warm smoothie if desired, only to touch.

Note: If you would like it to be thicker add less water or if you want it more liquidy add more water.

AVOCADO SMOOTHIE

INGREDIENTS

3 Bananas
2 Dates
2 Cups of Baby Kale
3 Tbsp of Avocado
2 Cups of water

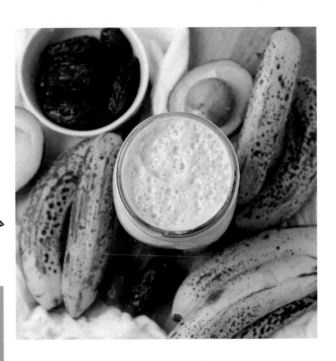

APPROXIMATE MICRONUTRITION BREAKDOWN

Total Calories: 535
Total Fat: 8.5g
Total Protein: 6.8g
Total Carbs: 122.4g

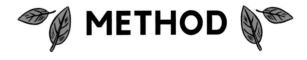 **METHOD**

In a high speed blender, blend all the ingredients until smooth. Warm smoothie if desired, only to touch.

Note: *If you would like it to be thicker add less water or if you want it more liquidy add more water.*

CUCUMBER SUNRISE

INGREDIENTS

1 Cucumber
2 Cups Baby Kale
1 Lemon Juice
1 Cup Parsley
6 Dates
2 Tbsp of Avocado
2 Cups of water

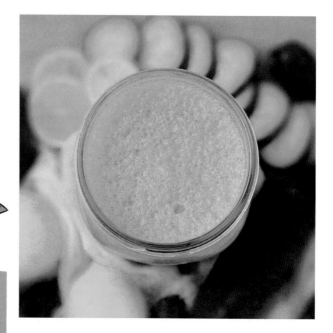

APPROXIMATE
MICRONUTRITION BREAKDOWN

Total Calories: 540
Total Fat: 6.2g
Total Protein: 8.6g
Total Carbs: 130.8g

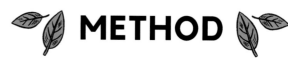 **METHOD**

In a high speed blender, blend all the ingredients until smooth. If you want this drink warm, only warm it to touch.

Note: If you would like it to be thicker add less water or if you want it more liquidy add more water.

V8 SMOOTHIE

INGREDIENTS

1 Handful of Parsley
2 Tomatoes
2 Cups of Spinach
2 Stalks of Celery
1 Carrot
5 Dates
2 Cups of water

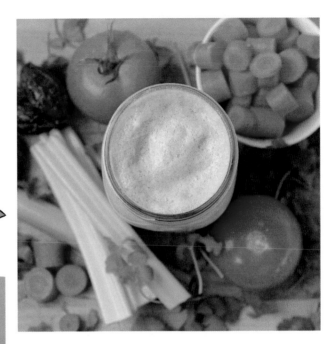

APPROXIMATE MICRONUTRITION BREAKDOWN

Total Calories: 518
Total Fat: 5.0g
Total Protein: 11.6g
Total Carbs: 122.5g

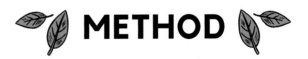 **METHOD**

In a high speed blender, blend all the ingredients until smooth. Add 1 Tbsp of chia seeds to smoothie after you blend.

Note: *If you would like it to be thicker add less water or if you want it more liquidy add more water.*

PITAYA PASSION FRUIT

INGREDIENTS

1 Frozen Pack of Dragon Fruit
2 Cups of Mixed Greens
4 Bananas
2 Cups of water

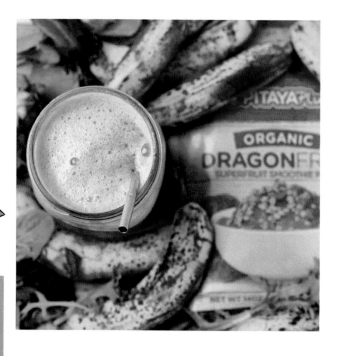

APPROXIMATE MICRONUTRITION BREAKDOWN

Total Calories: 548
Total Fat: 4.9g
Total Protein: 9.5g
Total Carbs: 128.6g

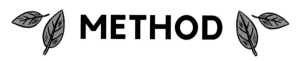 **METHOD**

In a high speed blender, blend all the ingredients until smooth. Add 1 Tbsp of chia seeds to smoothie after you blend.

Note: *If you would like it to be thicker add less water or if you want it more liquidy add more water.*

CINNAMON DATE SHAKE

INGREDIENTS

2 Bananas
4 Dates
1 Tbsp of Cinnamon
2 Cups of water

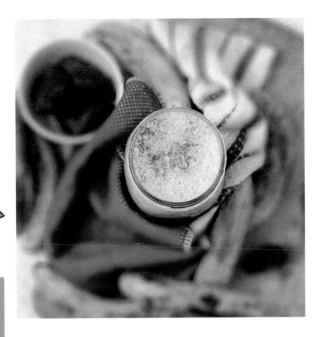

APPROXIMATE
MICRONUTRITION BREAKDOWN

Total Calories: 544
Total Fat: 4.1g
Total Protein: 6.3g
Total Carbs: 136.4g

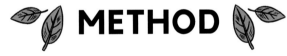 **METHOD**

In a high speed blender, blend all the ingredients until smooth. Add 1 Tbsp of chia seeds to smoothie after you blend.

Note: *If you would like it to be thicker add less water or if you want it more liquidy add more water.*

GREEN CHOCOLATE

INGREDIENTS

4 Bananas
2 Cup of Spinach
1 Tbsp of Cacao Powder
2 Cups of water

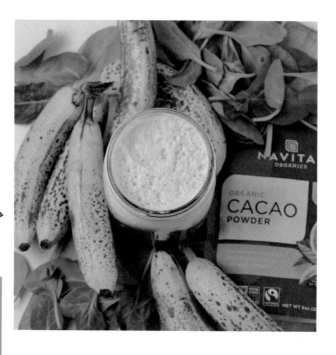

APPROXIMATE MICRONUTRITION BREAKDOWN

Total Calories: 543
Total Fat: 6.4g
Total Protein: 12.5g
Total Carbs: 123.2g

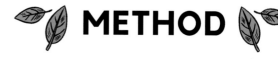 **METHOD**

In a high speed blender, blend all the ingredients until smooth. Add 1 Tbsp of chia seeds to smoothie after you blend.

Note: *If you would like it to be thicker add less water or if you want it more liquidy add more water.*

GREEN WARRIOR

INGREDIENTS

1 Tbsp of Flaxseed
2 Cups of Baby Spinach
4 Bananas
2 Cups of water

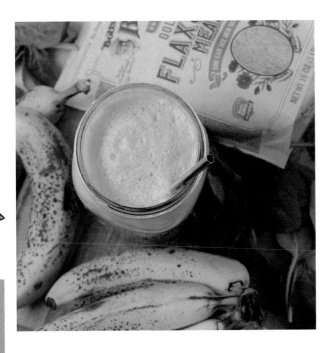

APPROXIMATE MICRONUTRITION BREAKDOWN

Total Calories: 576
Total Fat: 5.1g
Total Protein: 9.4g
Total Carbs: 139.0g

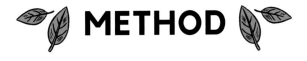 **METHOD**

In a high speed blender, blend all the ingredients until smooth. Add 1 Tbsp of Flaxseed to smoothie after you blend.

Note: *If you would like it to be thicker add less water or if you want it more liquidy add more water.*

THANK YOU!

Thank you so much for supporting me and allowing me to do what I love. It was my pleasure to make this book as so many people wanted to know how I did this challenge.

Thank you for choosing more raw foods into your diet, you are making the perfect choice for you to have a better life.

Continue to follow me on social media for more of my raw lifestyle.

Instagram: @RawndaFlowers
Website: RawndaFlowers
YouTube: RawndaFlowers
Pinterest: RawndaFlowers
E-Books: payhip.com/RawndaFlowers